General View Of The Agriculture Of The County Of Bedford: With Observations On The Means Of Improvement...

Thomas Stone

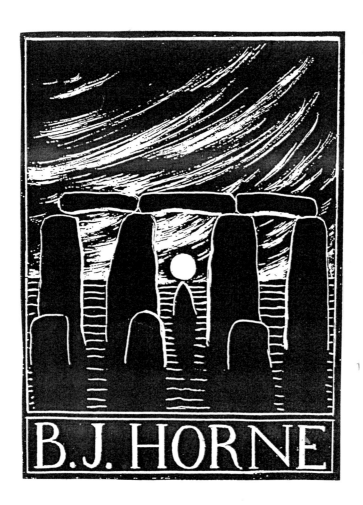

B.J. HORNE

GENERAL VIEW

OF THE

AGRICULTURE

OF THE

COUNTY OF BEDFORD;

WITH

OBSERVATIONS ON THE MEANS OF IMPROVEMENT.

BY

THOMAS STONE,

LAND SURVEYOR, GRAY'S-INN.

DRAWN UP FOR THE CONSIDERATION OF
THE BOARD OF AGRICULTURE AND INTERNAL IMPROVEMENT.

London:
PRINTED BY E. HODSON, BELL-YARD, TEMPLE-BAR

1794.

Entered at Stationers Hall.

TO THE READER.

It is requefted that this paper may be returned to THE BOARD OF AGRICULTURE, at its office in *London*, with any additional remarks and obfervations which may occur in the perufal, *written in the margin*, as foon as may be convenient.

It is hardly neceffary to add, that this report, is, at prefent, printed and circulated, for the purpofe merely of procuring farther information, refpefting the hufbandry of this diftrift, and of enabling every one, to contribute his mite, to the improvement of the country.

The BOARD has adopted the fame plan, in regard to all the other counties in the united kingdom ; and will be happy to give every affiftance in its power, to any perfon, who may be defirous of improving his breed of cattle, fheep, &c. or of trying any ufeful experiment in hufbandry.

LONDON, JULY, 1794.

INTRODUCTION.

AGREEABLY to the orders of the BOARD of AGRICULTURE, communicated to me by SIR JOHN SINCLAIR, its Prefident, I have undertaken to defcribe, in as concife terms as the extent of fo interefting a diftrict will admit of, the prefent ftate of the Agriculture of the county of BEDFORD; in the progrefs of which defign, fhould any of my ftatements feemingly bear too hard upon the conduct or management of particular individuals, it is not intended by me as any perfonal reflexion upon them. The faithful execution of the important bufinefs committed to my charge, muft at any rate, fuperfede every other confideration : And in whatever inftances I may commit errors, the fubject (from the plan fo happily adopted by the Board, of circulating thefe reports previous to their being publifhed) lies open to after-difcuffion, correction, and improvement. It muft occur, alfo, to the mind of every perfon of obfervation, and candour, that the bufinefs of a reformer is an arduous tafk, and attended with innumerable difficulties to execute it to advantage, when even a fingle object is in view; but becomes ftill more arduous, when a variety of points are to come under difcuffion.

Every country has its excellencies and defects, as well in the inherent qualities of its foils as in the manners, cuftoms, and modes of management of its inhabitants. And it behoves thofe perfons, whofe province it is, whether as proprietors, agents, ftewards, or otherwife, to correct mifmanagement and exifting abufes, in any particular parifh or diftrict, to be well afcertained of the practicability, and the probable advantages, to be derived from fubverting, or altering

any

any abuses, before they set out upon the measure. If that point be not strictly attended to, any miscarriage necessarily tends to bring a very unfortunate degree of discredit upon many other procedures, the success of which would be certain; thereby casting a damp upon the progress and the spirit of improvement.—It is no less necessary to examine strictly into the implements of husbandry, and to compare them with their uses, that no advantages may be overlooked, and a less applicable sort substituted for a better: Such circumstances have happened, where a violent zeal for reformation has ran before every other consideration. On the other hand it is to be observed, that every occupier of land, whose knowledge and pursuits have been confined to any given parish or district, has formed to himself an idea of that mode of management, upon the soil he occupies, which appears to him the utmost point of perfection; and he pursues it in a more or less direct path, in proportion to his capital, his permanency in his situation, and a variety of indirect views, will allow him. When any question shall arise upon the annual value of such his occupation, he does not scruple to stand up with confidence, and assert, (what he verily believes to be true), that he knows the value of it better than any other man; he has sown and reaped upon it, he has seen it in every season for a series of years:—And the plausibility of such assertions very frequently have weight, with persons of great good sense and abundant knowledge of the world. In vain might any person who has made agriculture his particular study, and who might be versed in the best modes of husbandry, of all the improved counties, come forth to inform him, that his mode of managing his farm tends to continue the soil weak and foul; that he too often ploughs it, and crops it with white grain: that meliorating crops should be interwoven therewith, and that it should be laid down with the first crop of corn, sowing grass seeds, next after a fallow, and turnips, for two or three years: that lime would be a

considerable

confiderable improvement upon the foil, which perhaps is cheap, and at hand: That a confiderable portion of meadow land might be flooded at pleafure, according to the Somerfet-fhire plan of making water meadows: That upon fearching into the bowels of the earth there is a probability of finding marle, or clay, which would greatly tend to fertilize the fur-face, if judicioufly laid upon it, together with innumerable other improvements which might be pointed out: whilft an-cient prejudices remain, the moft convincing arguments are ineffectual. It is example, and the imitation of it enforced by gentlemen of landed property, in particular their attention to the conditions on which their eftates are poffeffed, and that only, that can bring about a radical cure.

Thefe general obfervations being premifed, we fhall now proceed to the more immediate object of this Report.

GENERAL

GENERAL STATE.

THE COUNTY OF BEDFORD, though fo near the metropolis, is not remarkable for the excellence of its agriculture or attention to its breeds of cattle or fheep. The climate is mild and genial, and favourable to the growth of corn or vegetables. Its furface is diverfified by the hills and vales, and by nature, there is no diftrict in the ifland better adapted for improvements.

The principal river is the Oufe which runs acrofs the county from the Buckinghamfhire fide, through the town of Bedford to St. Neots in Huntingdonfhire. The Ivel empties itfelf into the Oufe at Tempsford; befides which rivers are the Lea and other fmaller ftreams of no confiderable importance.

The extent of this county is computed at 35 miles from North to South, and 20 miles from Eaft to Weft, and 145 miles in circuit, containing an area of 480 fquare miles or 307,200 acres, divided into nine hundreds comprifing 124 parifhes with 10 market towns (viz.) Bedford, Woburn, Ampthill, Bigglefwade, Dunftable, Leighton-Buzzard, Luton, Potton, Shefford, and Tuddington.

Agriculture, Manufactures and Commerce have made but very narrow ftrides towards the population and improvement of this county, the making of thread lace forms the principal part of the manufactures; the chief importation is coals for fuel and blackfmith's work, deals, fir, timber and falt; its exports are fuller's earth, oak-timber, and corn; the latter commodity is chiefly vended by the growers on the North

part

part of the county at St. Neots in Huntingdonfhire, and on the South and Eaft at Hitchin in Hertfordfhire, fo that except in the town of Bedford, very little bufinefs is done in the corn trade, and with regard to feveral of the other towns very little more than the name of market remains. Before a dreadful fire which happened a few years ago at Potton, that town poffeffed a very flourifhing market for corn, &c. but fince that time, it has not been much reforted to.

Of the 307,200 acres contained in this county, from the beft information I have been able to obtain upon the fubject, it may be computed that 68,100 acres are inclofed meadow, pafture and arable land; 21,900 acres of woodland, and 217,200 acres of open or common fields, common meadows, commons and wafte lands.

Upon a view of the neglected ftate of the agriculture of this diftrict, by a perfon acquainted with the improved agriculture of many other parts of England on fimilar foils, and who fhould be unacquainted with its geographical fituation, he would naturally conclude, that inftead of its centre being not more than 50 miles from the metropolis, that it was 500. Inftead its being defirably circumftanced in having a navigable river running from its centre to the ocean, poffeffing alfo almoft every other advantantage which nature or art * could give it for exporting or converting its produce to the greateft advantage, he would rather conclude, that it was inacceffible by means of bogs and barriers, and that its produce had no other market than that which arofe from the mere confumption of its inhabitants.

It will be expected as a matter of courfe, that as I have the honor of being called upon to reprefent in the beft manner in my power, the prefent ftate of the agriculture of this county, that I fhould alfo give my ideas of the caufe of the

---

* I fhall hereafter have occafion to mention, a profpect of great advantage, in a junction of the Oufe at Bedford, with a branch of the Grand Junction Canal.

neglected

neglected condition of the interests of the land-owners, the occupiers, and the community in this respect, and to suggest an adequate remedy.—Impressed with a due sense of the honor the Board of Agriculture has been pleased to confer upon me I proceed to suggest:

That one principal cause of this delay in the improvement of the agriculture of this county, has been the inattention, which, till of late, gentlemen of landed property, have shewn towards advancement in rural œconomy, and to improvement in a science in which they are so materially interested.

The frequently committing the management of their country concerns into the hands of persons, who are totally unacquainted with agriculture, or, in other words, considering that one and the same person, who receives and pays with great integrity, is equally competent to suggest or enforce improvements in the uses or prevent abuses in the management of land, whilst, in fact, with the same propriety might a mere husbandman be called from the plough, to amputate a limb, in the expectation of his having the skill of an experienced surgeon, or a seaman be directed to draw a marriage settlement, with the technical accuracy, and legal knowledge, of an experienced conveyancer. Hence it is that the dividing and inclosing mixed property, regulating the husbandry which ought to be observed upon it; the granting leases with a view to enforce the application of the most approved methods which ought to be adopted upon the different soils, and thereby securing the occupier in the enjoyment of the fruits of his skill, industry, and first expence, together with the compatible improvement of the inheritance in the land, and many other advantages of great moment hereafter to be enumerated, have not been adopted.

SOILS.

SOILS.

EVERY foil and every mixture of foil, commonly feen upon high land in the united kingdoms, may be found in this county, from the ftrongeft clay to the lighteft fand.

The property of the refpective proprietors in which, is mixed in the common fields generally in the fame way, with but little variation in point of management. In the North and Weft parts, clayey and ftrong loamy land moft prevails, on the South and Eaft we find mixed, light loamy, fandy, gravelly, and chalky foils*. For the fake of making myfelf the better underftood, it is my intention to reprefent the mode of management now practifed upon the refpective foils with fome fuggeftions of the means which I conceive neceffary to be adopted for their improvement.

* When I began to infpect the land it was my intention to reprefent by a map, the mixtures and connexions of different foils, but having upon experiment frequently found that one and the fame parifh produced four or five different foils, nothing but a particular furvey could have anfwered the purpofes of delineation, which would have been foreign from the prefent defign.

OF

OF STRONG LOAMY AND CLAYEY SOILS.

THE common fields of thofe defcriptions of foils, are generally divided into three parts, feafons, or fields, one of which is annually fallowed, a moiety of which fallow field (according to the beſt mode of management) is annually folded with ſheep and fowed with wheat, the other moiety of ſuch fallowed land is dunged and fown with barley in the fucceeding fpring, and that part which produces wheat is in fucceffion fown with oats, that which is next after fallow fown with barley, is in the fucceeding year fowed with beans, peas, or other pulfe, and then fuch land being again to be fallowed, that part which in the previous courfe of hufbandry was fown with wheat, comes in rotation to be fowed with barley, by which procedures the fame kind or fort of grain is only produced every fixth year. The foregoing is the beſt practice of the common fields upon this defcription of foil, but it is too frequently infringed upon by felf-interefted or ſhort-fighted farmers, or thofe who are preparing to depart from their occupations, and too large portions of land are fown with wheat and oats, fo that the rotation of cropping upon fuch land, comes round every third year, by which procedure and the repetition of the fame kind or forts of grain (and thofe of the moſt impoverifhing natures) the foil becomes exhaufted and foul, and thus all (but moſt particularly) thin ſtapled foils, are rendered unproductive, and cannot be brought into their former ſtate of fertility, under the beſt mode of common field management for a feries of years.

It is a common practice, to make open water furrows, and fuperficially to drain this defcription of land, when crops of

corn

corn are fowed, or in the firſt ſtages of their growth, but attempts of the like nature are very ſeldom made at other ſeaſons, from which negleƈt, the fineſt particles of manure, mucilage, or food for plants, are waſted or waſhed away, and the cells of the plants are rotted, and conſequently their tubes are either waſted or deſtroyed. The like inattention prevails with re-ſpeƈt to the draining of the commonable land, appendant upon ſuch common fields, from which circumſtance, not only ſimi-lar effeƈts in a ſmall degree are produced with reſpeƈt to the loſs of manure, and delay of the vegetation, but the deſtruc-tion of cattle depaſtured thereon is but too frequently pro-duced, and particularly the rot in ſheep, a diſorder about the immediate cauſe of which, although the ſkilful are apt to differ, yet all agree, that it is moſt likely to be contraƈted in wet ſeaſons and ſituations, where water is partially confined upon graſs land in furrows, and other low places.

Land of the foregoing deſcription (*i. e.* of a clayey nature) whether in a ſtate of arable or paſture, has been evidently ridged up for a ſeries of years upon a falſe principle of drain-ing 'till the tops of the ridges for ſix or eight feet acroſs are the only profitable parts of the ſoil;—the land next to, and the furrows form ſo many pools, ditches, and reſervoirs of water.

To level haſtily, land thus accumulated into heaps, would be a means of bringing ſo much dead earth upon the ſurface, that an occupier's intereſt in the whole of the land would be very materially delayed for three, ſix, or nine years, a circum-ſtance as to delay of intereſt which would ill agree with the condition of an occupier for only a round of cropping *.
There are but few inſtances in this county where the arable

---

* It may not be here improper to remark, that the occupiers of common field farms, as tenants at will, are entitled to hold poſſeſſion for a round of crop-ping, according to the number of ſeaſons, upon this ſort of land (where it is farmed in three years) and an ejeƈtment will not lie upon the common notice to quit at the end of a year.

land

land is divided into four fields or feafons, and where it is fo circumftanced, nothing like fyftem prevails, and the occupiers are generally at liberty to exhauft the foil at pleafure.

Upon inclofed arable and pafture of this defcription, the fame fhort-fighted, felf-interefted, or injudicious mode of farming is frequently practifed ; repeated crops of white grain, a general rejection of the beft mode of cultivating of green food, (fuch as turnips, cole, or cabbages), from an idea of the land being too wet to produce either, or a general neglect in not properly preparing the land for their production, or in not fowing or fowing or planting them in due feafon, and afterwards not properly hoeing them, and almoft a total neglect of the following improvements, viz. The keeping the main ditches fufficiently deep and open under the fences—The making funnels at the gateways—The competently conveying the water to a proper outfall—The properly plafhing and then guarding the young fhoots of the quick fences from fheep—The hollow draining of fprings and preventing the lodgment of water on the furface—The levelling of ant-hills—The cleaning the pafture land from bufhes and coarfe foul productions—The rolling it at fpring and autumn with an heavy roller—The neglect of the drill-hoeing and dib-bling-hufbandry, where thefe operations are refpectively practicable—The applying of manure which ought (under the moft profitable mode of occupation) to be laid upon the pafture land to the forcing white grain crops.

And laftly—Where there is a mixture of arable or pafture lands in the hands of one and the fame occupier, the not adopting fuch a mode of occupying the arable part, by inter-weaving meliorating crops, between crops of white grain, whereby a part of the annual fupply of manure might be fpared from the arable to be laid upon the pafture, and thereby improving the whole of the occupation : Inftead of which, it is a frequent practice that every atom of manure which can be fcraped together is laid upon the arable to force white
straw

ſtraw grain crops, which are produced as long as the ſoil will make any return for ſeed and labour, it then becomes weak, poor and foul, and the proceſs of fallowing is again reſorted to as the laſt reſource to reſtore it.

The paſture land not being manured is here devoted to every poſſible reduction of condition, the drainage is moſtly neglected, poached up in winter, and ſuffered to be over-run with ant-hills, buſhes, ruſhes and ſedge, and in many inſtances repeatedly mown.

Would a valuer of eſtates do juſtice to a landowner who was about to ſell his property, if he was to conſider ſuch land with reſpect to its *preſent condition only?* or as to ſuch reaſonable and practicable improvements of which it might be capable?—Much leſs on a contemplation of ſuch improvements ought thoſe to be rejected, or laid aſide, which can eaſily be brought about without any extraordinary labour or expence.

D   MIXED

MIXED SOIL, GRAVELLY, CHALKY, AND LIGHT LOAMY SOILS.

———————————

THE common fields of thefe defcriptions of foil are generally underftood to be divided into three, and in a few inftances four, parts or feafons, and here turnips are fown upon
confiderable parts of the fallow land, which are fucceeded by
barley fown with clover, which clover remains one year for
a crop, and is fometimes faved for feed, and the fourth crop is
generally wheat; but where there are but three fields, the
crop of clover is confidered as a breach crop inftead of beans,
peas, or oats, and the land which produces clover, is in fucceffion fallowed, and that apportionment intended for barley is
firft fowed with turnips; but thefe practifes are not purfued
fyftematically; the occupiers not being generally confined to
any particular modes of farming, follow fuch methods as feem to
promife them the moft immediate gain, without any direct view
to the future. The major part of the occupiers in each parifh being tenants from year to year, or, for a round of cropping, and not having any permanency in the occupation of
the foil, or from other caufes, want an incitement or encouragement towards the introduction of improved agriculture,
which can only be infpired by judicious leafes enforcing the
moft approved practical hufbandry, brought about by the fepa-
ration of the prefent combined, and mixed ftate of the open
common fields, common meadows, commons, and wafte lands,
by means of dividing and inclofing. Whilft the prefent
mode of occupying the foils remain, both the fpirit for, and
the means of exertion are dormant, nor are the occupiers generally

nerally advocates for an alteration of the property by means of inclofing and dividing it, for if they can get their bread in their prefent mode of farming, they are apprehenfive that they might not do more in cafe a general alteration of the condition of the property was to take place, not being acquainted with the improved agriculture which ought to take place upon an in- clofure ; and from a prejudice generally grafted in their minds againft innovations, or alterations, they do not readily change into new fyftems of farming, even where the benefit of ex- ample is immediately before them ;- unlefs the very condition of their holding is interwoven with the beft practice which can be adopted, and fecured by means of leafes properly drawn in conformity with improved hufbandry (before alluded to) and vigoroufly carried into execution under the fuperintend- ance of competent agents.

A general neglect of agricultural improvements in the let- ting of farms, and in the general unfkilful mode of raifing rents whenever the meafure is fet about, has brought the far- mers to apprehend that whenever they fhall difcover a fpirit for improvements, and in any degree put them in practice, a fpeculation would be made upon their exertions, and thus they might pay a fecond time for their improvements. The confequences attending the mode of raifing rents (before al- luded to) may be thus explained.

The tenant's holding being from year to year, or for a round of cropping, of courfe they cannot be faid to have any permanency in their refpective occupations, and in fome in- ftances are thus kept in conftant jeopardy. If a few flatter- ing feafons prefent themfelves, they are led to expect an ad- vance of rent, and except in tenancies under fome old, noble and refpectable families they are feldom baulked in their ex- pectations, and whether fuch additional rent is a light or an heavy burthen, the farmers are led to confider it as fo much wrefted from their hard earnings. No material improvements. or profitable alterations of the property being fuggefted on

the

the part of the land-owner, whereby the occupier might be benefited or amply repaid; and it is a matter of accident that it was not heavier.

A little more rapacity on the part of the land-owner, harder hearts, or softer heads on the parts of of the surveyors or agents employed, might have made it intolerable. A repetition of the like conduct in the land owner drives the occupier to despair, destroys all confidence on his part, and every degree of spirit being thus repressed, the tenantry carry on the business of their occupations as if they were constantly under notices to quit: In vain may the land-owner issue forth his assurances that if hard times shall come and the produce of the land be thereby reduced in value, the rents shall be lowered; to carry this idea to the fullest extent or to the hinge upon which the evil turns, it is keeping the tenantry in a galling state of dependance, and preventing them from every possibility of enriching themselves by extraordinary labour, diligence, and skill, or by the expenditure of their hard earned modicum in improvements, from a want of a permanency in the soil and a certainty of being reimbursed with interest and advantage by means of leases.

The land-owner need not apprehend that by granting leases of his property he relinquishes any of the gentlemany appendages, and consequence attached to the possession of land, for when the course of husbandry and every necessary and practicable improvement shall be pointed out for so long as the demise shall continue, the leases may be made voidable by either party giving six months notice to the other. The spirit of improvement is not altogether to be inspired by the length of the term of a lease,—the lease may be made for a short term very desirably, if the allowances for the tenant's improvements are liberally considered when he shall quit possession; for instance—the lessor paying the lessee (in case he gave him notice to quit) certain stipulated allowances for such improvements which may have taken place since the

com-

commencement of the term ;—and in cafe the leffee gives the leffor notice that he fhall quit the poffeffion, certain matters and things of courfe muft be performed by him agreeable to the original ftipulations.

A plan of this fort for ftrengthening the affurances between landlord and tenant, and for promoting improved agriculture, though fhort of the utmoft good that might be obtained from proper leafes, yet in particular cafes would be infinitely more beneficial than the prefent flovenly, loofe, and unproductive mode of occupancy, by which the land-owner, the occupier, and the community are every day fuffering very confiderable loffes.

In a diftrict fo large as the county of Bedford there is certainly a diverfity of management both with regard to the interefts of landlord and tenant, and inftances may be adverted to where the land-owners are noblemen and gentlemen of the firft fortunes and higheft refpectability, purfue a line of conduct extremely fteady and liberal towards their tenantry, and on the other hand inftances occur where the occupiers approach nearer towards perfection than in others, neverthelefs but a fmall part of the land in this county is managed in conformity to the moft approved modes of agriculture which have long been practiced in the beft cultivated counties upon fimilar foils.

The inclofed eftates of the laft mentioned defcriptions of foil are generally managed in a manner proportionably unproductive of advantage with the common fields, and the only benefit they appear to derive from their ftate of feveralty is the readinefs with which they may be improved on account of fuch feveralty only ; the occupiers not having been bound to improved agriculture have not adopted the drill, or dibbling, or hoeing hufbandry, nor any regular fyftems of cropping the land, producing ameliorating crops, interwoven with white grain, thereby keeping up the heart and good condition of the foil independent of foreign aid.

The

The properly fallowing, cultivating and hoeing turnips, or other green winter food for cattle and sheep, such as cole or rape, and cabbages, and sowing artificial grass seeds with the succeeding crop of barley to remain laid down therewith for one or more years *, are objects in the pursuit of which the majority of the Bedfordshire farmers are near a century behind Norfolk and Suffolk. The soils upon the management of which I am now remarking, are the most profitable under judicious management, and the reverse when improperly treated.

Upon a due investigation it will be found, that these soils are seldom to be found clean, or even made so by the progress of fallowing, which business is here made subservient to all other occasional business upon a farm ; in the improved counties, all other business is subservient to it, and where it is considered as the foundation of the whole and each part of the succeeding course of husbandry.

Turnips are but indifferently hoed, or the cultivation of them generally neglected, so that 20s. to 3l. may be said (upon a moderate calculation) to be annually lost upon all the green vegetable winter crops, for want of due attention and management: instead of the land being laid down with the first crop of spring corn with good artificial grass-seeds for one or more years in order to bring it to a turf, before it shall be again brought into a state of cultivation, it is often sown with a second, and sometimes a third crop of white grain, and with such second or third crop in succession, red clover and rye grass is often sown, thus the land becomes poor, foul and consequently unproductive, and when brought into that state it is impossible but by means untried and unknown in this part of the country to get it into heart, for here, the chief dependence is upon the common stable or fold-yard manure,

* The sowing rye, tares, &c. upon the stubbles intended for the succeeding fallows for support of stock in the most trying season of the year, which is that immediately after turnips, cole, or cabbages are exhausted, and before the natural or artificial grasses are ready.

which

which decreafes in the fame ratio as the land declines in its product.

The benefit to be derived from a judicious application of marle, clay, or lime, are, as I before obferved, generally unknown, the plodding upon the fuperftratum of five or fix inches content the occupiers, they rarely fearch into the foil deeper, and for want of a permanency, a fixed term of years or competent affurances in their occupations, they have no fpirit to adopt expenfive improvements, in the refult of which, whatever benefits might prefent themfelves, they are apprehenfive that the land-owners would reap the moft material advantages;

I am as great an enemy as any man to the racking up the rentals of farms beyond a fair yearly value, and wherever the beft mode of agriculture is adopted and the beft and moft fuitable ftock of cattle and fheep are produced, or in other words wherever any given fpot is made as productive as it can poffibly be, the land-owner ought to be careful that he does not require a greater rent than the occupier can live well under and pay with chearfulnefs, referving the intereft of his money employed in bufinefs at leaft, and a fair gain for his fkill and perfonal exertion. It is the groveling, prejudiced, unfkilful, obftinate farmer that I point at, who rents his land at half the real value, and therefore exerts but half his induftry, great part of which is employed in endeavouring to conceal from the land-owner or his agents the real ftate of his property, and who carefully turns his face afide from any improvements leaft his landlord fhould reap a part of the fuccefsful advantages to be derived from them.

Here a field prefents itfelf in which a judicious furveyor, or agent, may exercife his fkill, judgement, and integrity, to the advantage of both landlord and tenant, as well as that of the community, by pointing out the various means of improvement of which the refpective foils are capable, giving the tenantry the power of carrying them into execution, and a

security

security in a competent term to be allowed them, or assurances equal thereto, whereby they shall reap the fruits of their labour, and uniting the interest of the landlord and tenant for their mutual benefit with a view to an improvement of the inheritance in the land, making the soil produce the utmost it is capable of, thereby promoting the general good of the community.

COMMONS

COMMONS IN PASTURE.

THERE are not any extensive commons of this description in the county, and those which remain, are mixed with, or appendant on the common fields, and are held according to the antient system of farming, as necessary for the depasture of of sheep, in order to fold upon the arable common fields.

INCLOSURES.

FROM the statement I have already made, of the large quantity of land, yet remaining in a state of common and arable fields, common meadows, and waste lands, it must appear, that very little land has been inclosed of late years; every parish which is commonly understood to be open, consists of a certain portion of antient inclosed land near the respective villages, but that proportion, compared with the open common fields in each respective parish, does not on an average exceed one tenth of the whole.

E   COMMON

COMMON FIELDS.

———

Of late years several common fields have been inclosed, but such parishes have not been selected for that purpose, with a direct view to improved agriculture; for in several instances, inclosures have been made of some of those common fields, of which improvement is the least certain, being a thin staple of soil upon very strong loamy and clayey land, whilst in several instances, the same proprietors of such common fields were also proprietors, or much interested in the improvement of other open common field parishes of mixed soil, and light loamy natures, the improvement of which, by means of inclosing, would have been certain.

I must confess myself to be at a loss to account, for this extraordinary delay of public and private benefit, and I can only further observe upon it, that most of such inclosures, must have been brought about, from motives not strictly combined with views to improved agriculture.

In but few instances, have we seen improved systems of farming, adopted upon the new inclosures which have taken place, and except Lidlington, the property of the Earl of Upper Ossory; Sundon, the property of Sir John Buchanan Riddell, Baronet, and Potton; it does not appear, that any regular systems of farming, were laid down upon the inclosing of land, or have been since pursued upon it; but it has been a practice for the persons who were the tenants in the open field state, to take the new inclosed land at a considerable advance of rent, without any knowledge of or view towards improved agriculture, and generally

nerally without any falutary reftri&ions as to managèment, or any example or encouragement towards good hufbandry. No wonder that fuch tenants purfued profpe&ts of immediate gain, without any view to future advantage; the land was cropped fucceffively with the moft exhaufting crops, it became poor and foul, and fuch proceedings have brought the meafure of inclofing very undefervedly into difrepute in this county.

The town of Bedford is chiefly furrounded by common fields, the foils of which are of the moft improveable nature by means of inclofing, whereby the barbarous pra&tices of the common fields might be abolifhed, and the foil applied fuc-cefsfully to the purpofes of improved cultivation. On ac-count of the vicinity to the town, the land might be laid down in pafture and applied to the fupport of trade and com-merce, neverthelefs the inhabitants are under the neceffity of travelling over the arable common fields, now let at from 12s. to 18s. per acre, to inclofed pafture land in other parifhes, at a much greater diftance, and of lefs intrinfic value, where they rent it from 2l. to 3l. per acre; and other inftances of a fimi-lar nature might be adverted to.

NEAT

NEAT CATTLE.

THE cattle bred in this county, are for the most part of a mixed kind, differing, according to various mixtures, from the Holderness, Lancashire and Leicestershire to the Alderney forts, and as it has not been a general practice, to attend nicely to the breeding from the best of any particular forts, we find them of a very inferior nature, but most particular with regard to their intrinsic value of feeding for beef, *after the first intention for the dairy is over*, a circumstance, which it is presumed ought to be weighed by those breeders, who are desirous of making the greatest profit from their occupations. We generally find them large in their heads, bones and bellies, and coarse in their horns, throats and necks; narrow in their hips, plates, chines, shoulders and bosoms, and high in their rumps; and consequently, wanting that due width and symmetry of body, which carries with it the inherent aptitude to become fat, with a smaller portion of nutritious aliment, in a much less time, than would be required to render others marketable. From animals of the foregoing description, therefore, much less profit is derived to the grazier, than might be fairly computed upon, were more attention paid to the breed of cattle than at present. A considerable quantity of land, in the southern part of the county, is used for dairies, and butter is from thence consigned for the London market. In the middle and northern part, there is not so large a portion of land applied to the maintenance of cows as in the southern part, and that which is so applied, is divided between the dairy, and suckling calves for the London market, as well as for home consumption. The butter made in the south part of the county, is generally much

superior

superior in quality to that made in the central and northern parts, which I attribute to the degree of attention neceffary to be paid to the manufacturing it for the London market, for unlefs it was fent thither in a good ftate it would not be fold. Butter is now confidered fo much an effential neceffary of life, that a daily demand for a certain quantity muft conftantly prefent itfelf, and if the quantity being of a good quality is infufficient to fupply that demand, fuch as is of an inferior quality generally finds a market, and on this account it is very rare, except in gentlemen's houfes and fome few farm houfes where the women are remarkable for their cleanlinefs, to find any butter of the beft quality either winter or fummer. A general inattention to cleanlinefs, in making the dairies receptacles for meat in its different ftates, and various other family productions, greatly tend by their effluvia, to taint the milk and cream, to which may be added, the neceffary labour and attention, in the not daily fhifting the cream into fcalded clean veffels, and in not churning often enough. It frequently occurs, that the cellars and dairies in fmall farm houfes are one and the fame place—I recommend, that in the conftruction of farm houfes, the dairies fhould always be placed in fhaded fituations, and applied wholly for fuch purpofe, and free from the effluvia of the farm yards. If the managers of large families, and inhabitants of towns, poffeffed refolution enough for a few weeks, to reject all the butter offered to them, that was not perfectly fweet and good, a certain reformation would be made, in the wholefome and palatable qualities of this article of conftant confumption.—But few calves are reared, and thofe made fat for veal, are generally of a very nice quality, and fent up from Bedford and many other towns in the county, killed and dreffed in provifion waggons, for the fupply of the London market; a reformation in this article I confider to be very practicable. It but too often occurs in the courfe of a fummer, that in very wet or tempeftuous wea-

ther

ther, the Thames becomes the receptacle of large quantities of meat thus conveyed to London, by which circumftance, not only the interefts of the parties immediately concerned, but that of the community are deeply injured. I fhould recommend an experiment, of making the bodies of provifion waggons, to convey in the fummer feafon the calves alive to London, whilft a frame might be conftructed over them, upon which to place hampers and bafkets of lefs perifhable provifion.

SHEEP.

SHEEP.

THEY are generally of a very unprofitable quality, but more especially thofe bred in the common fields, where the provifion intended for their maintenance, is generally unwholefome and fcanty; it is impoffible to give a defcription of any particular fort as the general breed of the county, becaufe jobbers are conftantly driving various forts from fair to fair, and felling them in the different counties, and from the undrained ftate of the commons and common fields, the ftock of fheep depaftured upon them, is but too frequently fwept away by the rot; and it being abfolutely neceffary, according to the prefent fyftem of farming, that their places fhould be conftantly fupplied with others for the folding of the land, under fuch circumftances of cafualty and neceffity, the healthinefs of the animal when purchafed, is the firft and almoft the only object of confideration with the farmers, with that view, fheep are purchafed by them of any country and of any defcription, the horned and polled are mixed together, and as a pretty general defcription of them I may venture to obferve, that they are coarfe in their heads and necks, proportionably large in their bones, high on the leg, narrow in their bofoms, fhoulders, chines and quarters, and light in their thighs, and their wool is generally of a very indifferent quality, weighing from three to four pounds per fleece. A few exceptions may be made to this defcription, in the fheep at Goldington, St. Leonard's, Ickwell, and a few other places, but generally fpeaking, upwards of nine tenths of the fheep of the common fields of the county, are of this defcription.

The sheep bred upon the inclosures, are generally of a much superior quality, being for the most part a mixture between the Lincolnshre and Leicestershire sorts, but they are not equal to the most perfect of either kinds, though very useful and profitable.

The weathers are generally sent to market from the inclosures when shorn twice, called *two shear*, and are sold when very fat at from 35s. to 40s. per head. Their fleeces generally weigh from seven to nine pounds each.

His Grace the Duke of BEDFORD, is making some very desirable experiments, in the comparative value of the different kinds of sheep, which will require some time, to reduce to that degree of critical accuracy, which a subject of so much general importance deserves.

Perhaps upon the republication of these observations, the public may be favoured from his Grace with some account of them.

Mr. BENNET, a farmer at Tempsford, upon the great north road, 52 miles from London, is possessed of a breed of that kind of sheep called the New Leicester, which do infinite credit to his judicious choice and perseverance to obtain, and it will require a very nice degree of judgment, to distinguish them, from those produced upon the land of some of the first breeders in Leicestershire.

From the experiments already made, upon the production of this truly valuable animal in this kingdom, and from the observations I have been enabled to make, the New Leicestershire breed, stands in the fairest light for pre-eminence, the smallness of their bones and offals, the width of their carcases, the abundant fineness of their fleeces, docility of temper, perfect symmetry of body, uniting with every other circumstance which can render them in the highest degree profitable, possessing that inherent quality of becoming fat with a much less portion of aliment than is requisite to keep alive sheep of a contrary description.

WOOD LAND.

THE improvement of this ſpecies of property, has not been much attempted, and it does not appear, that any material experiments have been made, in order to aſcertain the comparative advantages to be derived, from the cultivation of different kinds of timber and underwood, or in ſelecting ſuch ſorts as are beſt adapted for the moſt immediate uſes of the country. The woods or woodlands, conſiſt chiefly of oak timber and any kinds of rude underwood, that, by chance, may ſpring up under it, ſo that it is not unuſual, to ſee thorns produced, where a more valuable crop might be cultivated ; it not being an object of general attention at every fall of underwood, which is cut at about twelve or fourteen years growth, either to root out ſuch productions as are the leaſt profitable, and to fill up the vacant places with a better ſtock. It is not unuſual, to obſerve in the woods, conſiderable quantities of land, either quite vacant, or producing a ſmall crop of any thing ; indeed ſo inconſiderable is the crop of underwood, in the eſtimation of ſome perſons who have had the management of woods, that inſtead of felling the neceſſary timber at the time the underwood is cut, they have returned years afterwards to cut more timber, throwing it down upon ſuch of the young ſhoots of the underwood as were produced, which, if a tolerable crop, would be greatly injured by ſuch means, and alſo by the conveying it away.

The moſt profitable mode of managing wood-land, in my opinion, is to cultivate a regular quantity of ſuch kinds of

timber

timber and underwood together, as may be beft fuited to the foil, fituation and circumftances of the country where it may be produced. By this mode, the prefent generation, as well as pofterity, will be benefited.

This laft mode of managing wood-land, appears to me to have been generally neglected, and of late years, an object of lefs confideration in rural œconomy, than any other improvement. In the reign of HENRY the Eighth, we find feveral very falutary laws enacted, to prevent abufes in the management of wood-lands; probably fuch attention of the legiflature, might have been excited, by a general fpirit for cleanfing the ground of wood for cultivation, under an apprehenfion, that by converting fo much wood-land as was then intended to the purpofe of agriculture, the neceffary timber for the fupply of the navy would be too much diminifhed. From whatever caufe fuch reftrictions proceeded, the framers of them appear to have had a juft idea of the beft mode of cultivating wood-lands; by fixing the quantity of ftandrills to be left at every fall of underwood, it clearly appears to me, that the cultivation of underwood was confidered as a fixed object of profit, whilft the quantity of timber intended to be cultivated in fucceffion, appears to be the precife quantity, that might be raifed in the moft healthy and flourifhing ftate, without injuring the progrefs of improvement either in the underwood or timber, it being compatible with the raifing timber of fufficient height, and preferving to it that quantity of fpace, branch and foliage, fo neceffary for the admiffion of air, and the attraction of water and nourifhment from the atmofphere, for its health and fupport.

IMPROVEMENT

IMPROVEMENT

IN

TIMBER AND UNDERWOOD.

THE firſt thing which claims our attention is, a due inveſtigation, whether land, which is now uſed for the production of timber, is moſt profitably applied to ſuch purpoſe, under a due conſideration of the nature of the ſoil, and its local ſituation and circuſtances ? The ſecond, whether ſuch timber is adapted to the ſoil upon which it is produced? I am of opinion, that all land of an high quality, viz. from 18s. to 25s. per acre, might be moſt profitably applied to the purpoſes of cultivation; the advantages to be derived from an annual rent, produced from corn, graſs, &c. with its accumulating compound intereſt, will in a term of years, neceſſary for bringing a crop of timber to perfection, produce a much larger ſum than can be reckoned upon it.

Various calculations have been made, upon the probable advantages to be derived, from the cultivation of oak timber; but ſuch calculations are wholly founded on conjecture, as the probable term of human exiſtence falls ſo far ſhort of that length of time, which is neceſſary to bring this plant to perfection, upon ſoil the beſt adapted for its production, that regular, periodical, and competent obſervations, in particular inſtances, are loſt or hidden from our enquiries.

It

It is difficult to fet apart any fpot of land, as beft fuited for, the production of oak timber, which has not already produced it, becaufe fo much depends upon the fubftratums of foil, through which the tap root ought to find an eafy progrefs, in regular approaches towards perfection, and any inequalities, by means of ftony or hard bodies, which it may meet with in any ftage of its growth. I am of opinion, that all land of an high quality, that is to fay, from the yearly value of 18s. per acre and upwards, might be moft profitably applied to the purpofes of cultivation, the advantages to be derived from an annual rent produced from corn, grafs, &c. with its accumulating compound intereft, will, in a term of years neceffary for bringing a crop of timber to perfection, produce a much larger fum, than can be recovered upon it.

Particular inftances have occurred, where a large quantity of timber has been produced in high perfection, where the trees have been very thick with but little foliage ; but it has been in thofe fituations, where the foil is extremely deep and rich, making amends for the exclufion of a very confiderable part of the atmofpheric nutriment, which, on foils lefs fertile, is abfolutely neceffary to be imbibed by the plants for their health and fupport. If the oak has fpace for its branches to expand themfelves, fifteen trees, containing on an average from 80 to 100 feet of timber each, will cover an acre of ground. And unlefs, as in the cafe before ftated, the trees have fufficient room for the expanfion of their branches, their growth will be impeded in proportion as they are cramped. Thin ftapled clays of a low quality, fuch as are found in the weft part of Huntingdonfhire, and the high parts of Cambridgefhire, and north parts of this county, now let under ten fhillings per acre, are probably well adapted for the production of timber and underwood; and, upon the pooreft cold foils of this county (though the quantity is fmall), timber and underwood fhould be continued where found, and im-

proved

proved on land where it is planted, and fimilar foils might be converted into wood-land to great advantage.

It is impoffible that timber and underwood can be any where raifed, upon a given fpot, in a mixed ftate, in as large quantities, and to as much perfection, as they might be feparately; yet a very confiderable head of timber, may be raifed in fucceffion, with a good crop of underwood; and I confider this to be the moft profitable mode of employing fuch land, by which means, the prefent generation as well as pofterity may be benefited, and the land thus made much more productive than it would be, by the feparate cultivation of either timber or underwood, becaufe the fuperftratum may be fully employed in raifing the moft valuable crop of underwood; being that for which the foil is adapted; an advantage, which may probably be found applicable, to the neceffities of the country where it fhall be produced, and of a much higher net annual product for rent, than would be made of the land in any other mode of occupation; whilft the fubftratum is productive of a fucceffion of timber of confiderable value. I cannot clofe this remark without obferving, that the mode in which fome gentlemen permit their woods to be managed, is not the beft that can be devifed. I recommend that foreft officers, ftewards, agents, and woodmen, fhall have regular fixed falaries, and that they fhall not conftantly have it in their power to take advantage of their own wrong doing, for according to the prefent mode in fome inftances adopted, in the falling and converting timber, it is cuftomary for them to take part of the property in bark, topwood, &c. &c. or poundage as perquifites of office, upon the fale of it; and therefore, whilft the quantity annually to be cut is limited, and fuch officers are removed, it is their intereft not to cut down fuch trees as are mature or decaying, but otherwife the moft thrifty ones, which would, according to the beft modes of employing the land, pay moft for ftanding longer, as they will confequently produce moft bark, top or lopwood, and poundage.

FOLDING

FOLDING SHEEP.

I the neceffity for the meafure of inclofing common fields, commons, and wafte lands, and erecting competent conveniencies for farming the lands when inclofed, in central fituations, required any additional argument to thofe which have been commonly ufed—it might be adduced, from the univerfally acknowledged neceffity, of folding fheep upon a portion of fuch land annually; whereby in almoft every fituation, where this barbarous practice is adopted, the occupier throws away a much larger intereft, in the want of improvement in his fheep, than he gains by the manure he derives from their folding.

Wherever a foil is found fo poor, that it will not by being inclofed, and having farm houfes placed in central fituations, under a courfe of hufbandry beft adapted to the foil, afford animal and vegetable manure, in fufficient quantities, to keep it in good heart, without folding fheep upon it, I recommend its being thrown out of every agricultural view, and planted with that fort of timber, for the production of which it may be beft adapted.

DAIRY

DAIRY FARMING.

THIS mode of employing land, is of all others the moſt impoveriſhing, and more eſpecially upon cold or wet land, with a
clayey bottom, or where the ſuperſtratum is in any degree retentive of water, becauſe the poaching of the cattle, when the
land is in a wet ſtate, is extremely injurious to it. The neceſſity that there is alſo, for annually mowing a conſiderable
portion of it (at leaſt one-third) for the ſupport of cattle in
winter, to reinſtate which no manure can be afforded, is the
ſureſt means of reducing the value of the land. The only
ſituation in which a dairy can be ſupported to advantage, is
upon an incloſed farm, conſiſting of at leaſt one-third arable,
where the ſtraw-yard, or offals of turnips will maintain the
barren cattle, and the cows producing milk may be ſupported
upon turnips, and a portion of hay, as the circumſtances of
the occupation and neceſſities of the caſe will require; but
even in ſuch ſituations, two-thirds of paſture land, ſhould be
alternately ſtocked with ſheep, and ſuch beaſts as will eat off
the coarſe herbage.

FENCES.

FENCES.

———————

Notwithstanding the great care, attention, and expence, which is commonly employed in raifing new quickfet fences by the proprietors of eftates, how common a circumftance it is, to fee them afterwards totally neglected, or what is worfe, deftroyed by fubfequent bad management.

They are frequently fuffered to grow too long before they are plafhed, and when plafhed, to have live ftakes left in them, which afterwards fhoot out like pollard trees, whereby a confiderable part of the young fhoots, which fhould proceed from the ground, are thus mounted on ftilts, the hedges become thin at the bottom, and confequently, in a fhort fpace of time, fheep and other fmall animals creep through them.

The mode of cutting them is generally improper; indeed the whole fyftem of plafhing is badly performed, for in the firft inftance, the ftems of the quick are generally bent down and hacked nearly through, and laid into the hedges, which lets the water into the roots and decays them; they ought otherwife to be cut off at the bottom of the ftem with fharp inftruments, by ftrokes directed upwards, whereby the bottom of fuch ftems would be left fmooth and floping to fhoot off the water. It but too often occurs, that after fuch plafhings, the young fhoots are not properly protected from the biting of fheep and other animals.

I recommend, that whenever at 12 or 14 years growth, or at any times when the bottoms of the ftems of quickfet hedges

become

become thin, and lofe their bufhy productions, they fhould be wholly cut up in the manner before defcribed, and competently hedged or protected from the biting of cattle or fheep. It will but feldom occur, that the bufhes fo produced will do more than afford the means of hedging and defending the young fhoots, until they are paft being injured, &c.

Where fuch productions are incompetent, I recommend the ufe of ftrong fhifting hurdles, a good ftock of which fhould be provided by every farmer for this and various other ufeful purpofes.

RABBIT WARRENS.

THIS mode of occupying land, is very little practifed in this county, and is chiefly confined to two or three parifhes, where the production of the filver grey rabbit, is not attended to as in fome parts of Lincolnfhire, the fur of which fort is of a much higher value than that of the common grey rabbit.

PARING AND BURNING.

———————————

THIS species of management is but very little practised in this county. Indeed I know but one estate upon which it is now adopted, and there it is very limited in its extent. I observed that the land pared and burnt in the present spring is sowed with barley, the worst of all possible management.

In the Fens where this practice most prevails, the production of a green vegetable crop immediately after burning, is a common and a better practice; but here the farmer sets out with an exhausting crop, and there is no doubt of his going on with the same management, as long as a white straw grain crop can be produced—then when the soil shall become poor and foul, fallowing will be resorted to, as the only possible remedy, the manure arising from the crops so forced, will be applied to the forcing similar crops upon other land, until the whole will be quite exhausted at one and the same time, and then the means of restoring the soil to fertility, will be completely out of the farmer's power.

If the practice of paring and burning should at any time be absolutely necessary, in order to get rid of a variety of coarse productions, which cannot be subdued by any other means, (a circumstance which can hardly ever occur upon high land), I should recommend it ever afterwards to be abandoned, as a practice highly prejudicial to both the interests of landlord and tenant, for that soil which is already too light, requires not ashes to be mixed with it, the surest means of making it

lighter;

lighter; that soil which is already too thin or shallow, requires not to be subtilized with fire, the surest means of reducing its quantity. The ashes produced from burning the turf, are generally of a very forcing nature, and unless the soil upon which this practice is adopted, is frequently impregnated with large quantities of dung and mucilagenous substances, it soon becomes exhausted, and after a few years and the second stage of putrefaction has taken place, the effect produced, is the creation of salts of but little or no effect, or if they have any effect, they are hurtful to vegetation, and by this means the soil becomes a mere *caput mortuum.*

HORSES-

HORSES.

THE breeding of horfes is not a practice in this county worthy of particular obfervation, but few are bred except thofe defigned for pleafurable ufes.

The farmers teams are chiefly kept up, by yearling and two-years old colts, brought by dealers from the Fens of Huntingdon-fhire and Lincolnfhire. Some farmers practice the felling off their cart horfes for more valuable purpofes to profit at 6 or 7 years old, but the practice is not general. In the fouthern part of the county, where the farmers keep a road team to carry the produce of the land towards London, and to bring back London manure, fuch as fheeps trotters, horn fhavings, rabbits and fowls dung, &c. &c. fuch teams are kept very high, and of courfe at a very great expence; and I am of opinion (and which will be hereafter more particularly fhewn), that the farmers returns do not compenfate for fuch extra expence.

I recommend that every farmer fells off his working horfes according to the purpofes for which they are beft adapted, as they rife to fix and feven years old, and to fupply their places with young ones. Upon a moderate calculation, in refpect of the horfes employed upon an arable farm of 200l. per annum, for a term of twenty-one years, the difference between keeping a ftock of horfes conftantly improving and thofe declining in value, is at leaft 1000l.—A fimilar mode of felling off cows, or feeding them at fuch ages, would produce a proportionate benefit to the dairy-man or farmer.

I   FINES

FINES ARBITRARY, HERRIOTS, &c.

I recommend upon all inclofures and divifions of landed pro-perty, and in every other cafe where practicable, the enfran-chifement of copyhold eftates, from arbitrary fines, herriots, &c. for whilft the lord of a manor is entitled to two years improved value of them, upon the death of a copyhold tenant, or on the alienation of the property, particular cafes every day occur, to prevent the tenants from expending their pro-perty in the improvement of them.

THE

THE ROADS.

The public roads of this county, are generally speaking in a good state, but in some particular instances might be improved; the materials are for the most part good, and pretty regularly distributed.

The new roads are thrown up too round in the first instance before sound materials are laid upon them, by which procedure, the materials are much the thickest in the horse-path, and the strongest of them roll off the sides; there ought to be in the first instance a vacuum left in the middle of the road to deposit the strong materials in, as in the following figure:

If the Commissioners of the public roads were not only to cut down trees and clip hedges, but prevent trees being injudiciously planted by the sides of them, they would promote the public good.

The private or cross country roads are generally much neglected, and of course in a very bad state.

IMPROVE-

IMPROVEMENTS.

THERE are no focieties inftituted for the improvement of agriculture. The tenantry, who, for the moft part, are occupiers from year to year, have no incitement to exertions of fkill. The open ftate of the property, deprive them, in a great meafure, of the means of carrying improvements into execution; and at any rate, they want a certainty or fecurity, by means of leafes, for being reimburfed the expence of any improvements that might be confidered practicable; and they in general are fearful of fhewing any inclinations towards improvement, leaft a fpeculation fhould be made in an untimely, unqualified, and unjuftifiable advance of rent.

The only means of exciting a general fpirit for improvements, would be, by granting leafes under regulations to enforce the moft approved methods of agriculture, which are adopted with fuccefs upon foils of a fimilar nature, for gentlemen of extenfive landed property to fhew the way, by undertaking the occupancy of parts of their eftates, under the beft practical fyftems of Norfolk, Effex, Hertfordfhire, &c. &c. and the choiceft breeds of cattle and fheep to be found in England, rejecting experiments for a time, or leaving it for the active zeal of agricultural focieties.

ON

THE USE AND ABUSE OF LEASES.

———————

THE gentleman of landed property, who fhould make a refo-lution not to grant any part of his eftate upon a leafe, would commit as great an error as he who grants the whole in that way. There are but few eftates that are fo circumftanced as not to admit of improvement—few on which an occupier of abilities might not lay out a confiderable part of his property, for the fake of future advantages to his landlord as well as himfelf; on this account it is reafonable, that he fhould be fe-cured in his expectations as far human forefight will allow, and this is moft effectually done by a leafe. Though a gen-tleman's word may be as binding to him as his bond, his fuc-ceffor is not bound by it; therefore a farmer cannot be ex-pected to lay out his money, which is often the dependance of a family of children, upon the uncertainty of an occupation from year to year. Such gentlemen as are determined not to grant leafes at any rate, nor to give fuch affurances for the permanency of the occupier's intereft as may be relied upon, muft be content to let their eftates beneath their real value, and neglect many ufeful improvements, which would tend to their own, the tenant's, and the public advantage.

It is not an unufual thing for men of experience, to find eftates which are let much below their real annual value, in a much worfe condition than thofe which have been improved in point of yearly rent. We may fairly take the counties of

Norfolk

Norfolk, Suffolk, &c. for the examples in this respect, where a reasonable and proper advance of rent, with the leases of the property drawn out for the mutual advantages of landlord and tenant, giving the occupiers the means of using the soil to their utmost benefit, without abuse, has tended to the extreme opulence of the farmers. It is but reasonable, under such circumstances, that the soil should bear a rent, to enable the owner of it to purchase its product, according to the progressive decrease in the value of money.

Where an estate is let according to its yearly value, a lease is as necessary to secure a landlord's interest in the premises as the tenant's. Where a farmer occupies land from year to year, particularly arable lands, if he is self-interested, indolent, or injudicious, a farm may almost imperceptibly become impoverished before any alarm is taken; indeed such farms often fall into the proprietors hands in the most wretched condition. I have frequently heard gentlemen of landed property complain, that they are considerable losers by farming; and it may reasonably be accounted for, since the land usually comes into their hands in a reduced state, and in that case, let who will be occupier, two or three years rent must be sunk to restore it.

Rent is an annual sum paid by the tenant to the landlord, without diminishing the value of his property; and when the value of an estate is reduced by a bad or injudicious occupier, it cannot be called rent, but so much deducted from the real worth of the possession. Proprietors of land do not all of them consider this matter in a true light; and when they can advance the annual income of their estates, consider it as rent, whilst the property is often suffering in an equal proportion to the annual sum received during the demise, in at least an equal measure.

There are particular situations where long leases are unnecessary and improper, especially when farms consist wholly of rich pasture land, which will admit of no improvement; or

H   farms

farms lying near to gentlemen's feats or parks, where a difa-
greeable neighbour for a term of years would be a great inconvenience. But if gentlemen forego their own intereft and
that of the community, by not granting leafes, becaufe it
may poffibly be imagined that fuch tenants would become independent of their landlords, they are much miftaken; for
when leafes are properly drawn, it muft always be highly to a
tenant's prejudice to offend his landlord; fortuitous circumftances ever produce fome indulgence to be folicited from a
landlord; even exacting rent on the day it becomes payable,
would be an inconvenience which many tenants could not bear:
All farms fhould be let upon agreements, whether for one, or
twenty-one years, in a judicious manner, as near as poffible
for the mutual advantage of landlord and tenant, always preferving the value of the land; at leaft, wherever agreements
or leafes are not made with fuch views, or directed to fuch
ends, it would be better that no fuch leafes or agreements
fubfifted: though the value of the land would be likely to be
diminifhed, yet abufes would not be fo fpecioufly practifed, as
when they are admitted by ftipulated terms, reciprocally ef-
tablifhed between the proprietor and his tenant: Of this defcription are the common precedents of leafes, handed down
from one attorney to another, from a period before any improvements in the fcience of agriculture were adopted.

I cannot take leave of this fubject, without recommending it
to all gentlemen of landed property, as well as perfons defirous of hiring farms, to be cautious that farmers do not take
more land than their circumftances will admit of ftocking,
improving, and managing to the greateft advantage. Though
the ill confequences attending fuch practices both to landlord
and tenant are flagrant, yet they are but too frequent, by
which procedure many very induftrious farmers have been
ruined, and many eftates undefervedly brought into difrepute.

NEW

NEW PLANTATIONS.

In the western part of the county, the Earl of Upper Ossory, and Francis Moore, Esq. have, within the last twenty-five years, made some very considerable improvements, by planting light sandy land with trees.——Their plantations consist chiefly of mixtures of the fir tribe, and it appears, although in the outset, ornament engaged a considerable share of their attention, that such plantations have turned out extremely profitable. Mr. Moore has made some experiments upon the comparative value of the different sorts of plants, which he will doubtless communicate, with pleasure, to the Board of Agriculture.

I am of opinion, from the observations I have been able to make, that the Larch Fir is the most desirable tree to plant for profit, upon land of the foregoing description, in this county.

His Grace the Duke of Bedford is planting and beautifiyng many hundreds of acres of barren and waste land, in the neighbourhood of Woburn Abbey, which is laid out with great taste, and, I doubt not, will turn out, in every respect, beneficial.

Lord Carteret has raised some very ornamental plantations, near his seat at Haynes; and I am of opinion, that when the improvements, his Lordship is carrying on, are complete, nothing will remain upon his estate to be performed, which art can effect.

The

The practice of pruning timber and other trees, at various stages of their growth, is very prevalent in this county, as well as the making pollards of timber and timber-like trees. Whenever a tree, at any stage of its growth, has its branches lopped off, the body of it receives injury in a more or less degree, and, in proportion to its age and growth, it decays; but another injury, of no less consequence, is occasioned by robbing the trees of their branches and foliage, whereby the means of supplying them with moisture and nourishment is diminished. The injury is proportionably less, when practised upon very young trees; but, when timber, or timber-like trees, that have acquired thirty or forty years growth, suffer amputations, they immediately begin to decay, and when any very considerable quantity of branch and foliage are lopped off, such trees become bark-bound and stunted, and never more regain their former vigour. It may not be improper to remark, that every tree imbibes moisture from the atmosphere, impregnated with vitreous or other particles of manure, which greatly tend to nourish the plant; and if the foliage and branches, which serve to imbibe and conduct the moisture, thus impregnated with nourishment, to the root, where, according to the intention of nature, it should exsude or deposit a competent stock in reserve, are cut off, the means by which it should be supplied are thus crippled and diminished, decay of health is the consequence, and the plant ever afterwards is unthrifty and sickly.

It is very extraordinary, that in the present enlightened days, we should but too frequently observe the same hand, which is industriously employed in planting and watering a tree, afterwards destroying it, by pruning off its branches, and leaving a mere sprig on its upper branch, with only a few leaves upon it, merely to denote it is not quite destroyed. The most successful mode of planting trees, is to produce them very thick in the first stage of their growth, and afterwards to thin them judiciously at different periods, by which means, the trees will throw out very few branches on the sides of their stems, and

they

they will be carried up, if the foil is genial to their growth, to the moſt defirable height. The fuperfluous branches of young trees, are beſt rubbed off with an hedger's glove, in the feaſon in which they are thrown out. Crooked timber is very defirable for particular purpofes in the conſtruction of ſhips; and if his Majeſty's forefts will not, according to the preſent mode of managing them, fupply it with timber, it may be trained to grow crooked, to anfwer the fpecified purpofes for which it is required.

Thofe who cut off the tops of timber or timber-like trees, to make them what are commonly called pollards, have no excufe whatever to plead. This abominable practice gene-rally originates with neglect of the quickfet hedges, which, when fallen into decay, muſt be fupplied by dead ones, and in order to procure the neceffary materials, the farmer afcends the neighbouring trees, to lop off the neceffary materials; and in order to fecure a conſtant fupply of hedging ſtuff, he cuts off the leading branches, and afterwards claims the fuc-ceeding crop as his own.

THE

ON

THE PRODUCTION OF BEES-WAX AND HONEY.

THE means of producing the greateſt poſſible profit that can be derived from ſoil, cannot be completely purſued, until the production of honey and wax is fully attended to. Upon a moderate calculation, in which I have been affiſted by Mr. WILDMAN, of Holborn, a perſon, who has made this ſpecies of profit his particular ſtudy for many years—every ſquare mile in Great Britain, would produce in thoſe articles, on an average 100 l. ſterling in value, admitting that an increaſe of product would reduce the price of thoſe articles. But ſuch an increaſe in the quantity of bees-wax, would conſequently tend to render the importation, not only of thoſe articles, but of tallow, unneceſſary to the preſent extent. The value of theſe articles, on this ſtatement, far exceeds the idea of the moſt ſanguine friend to the proſperity of the country. There are in England alone, 49,450 ſquare miles, and in Scotland 27,794—total 77,244; which at 100 l. per ſquare mile, would produce 7,724,400 l. per annum. At only 20 l. per ſquare mile, the produce would be 1,544,880 l. This is an object well worth attending to, being in addition to every other profit derived from the ſoil.

If we examine the various purpoſes to which bees-wax is applied, it will, amongſt others, be found to be uſed in va-

rious

rious manufactures, in chirurgical and veterinary healings, and various family purposes. It is an article, in which luxury would be at a stand, unless it supplies the elegant and polite with light, to tread in almost all their nocturnal mazes, it aids in the construction of dress, and even the ladies apparel is impregnated with it. The medicinal uses of honey are universal; it is a luxury upon the table, and the best of all substitutes for butter and sugar; and when the finest particles are extracted, the refuse being properly converted into wine, when it becomes of a proper age and quite dry, is not inferior to the best of foreign white wine.

THE BEE.

THE advantages agriculture would derive from multiplying this industrious animal, are not few. By means of their industrious pursuits, in roving from blossom to blossom, the chives, or male parts, with more expedition and certainty, impregnate the pointels, which often, without such operation being expeditiously forwarded by such means (under a suspension in the want of air, or in consequence of violent rains), the seed is washed away before the intention of nature is performed, and the plants remain unfruitful.

THE

SWINE.

THIS animal, is not generally produced in as high perfection in this county, as in many others. The introduction of the beft forts from Berkſhire or Hampſhire, would be a very confiderable improvement.

POPULATION.

THERE not being any manufactures in this diſtrict deferving notice, agriculture is the only means of occupation; but from the uninclofed and uncultivated ſtate of the country, and the little employment and encouragement given to the huſband-men, in refpect to conſtant work throughout the year, the la-bourers continue with the farmers during the winter feafon, to thraſh out their grain, and on the approach of fummer, many of them fet off for more cultivated counties, where la-bour is more required; whereas, were a proper fyſtem of huſbandry introduced, thefe labourers would have conſtant employ in their own neighbourhood, and the number would be annually increafing. There is a fcarcity of comfortable cottages for the poor in this county; and the farmers are more ſtudious to prevent this very neceffary clafs of men from making fettlements among them, than to provide them ufeful and profitable employment.

THE

THE UNDERWOOD

Is not carefully selected and planted; the production of it, both in quantity and quality, is, for the most part, left to chance.

OAK TIMBER.

THIS species of wood is not produced in large quantities in this county, except upon the estate of his Grace the Duke of BEDFORD; nor is there a regular demand for that supply which the county affords; although there is a navigable river running to its centre. It is commonly purchased by jobbers in large lots, who generally convert it to any purposes by which a quick return can be had, with some immediate gain, and no scrupulous regard to the conversion of it to the purposes of ship building is had, a circumstance deserving of the attention of those most interested in the support of the navy.

I

IMPROVE-

IMPROVEMENTS

IN THE

AGRICULTURE OF THE COMMON FIELDS.

THE property of this defcription may be extremely improved, by being properly divided and made feveral; but a queftion always arifes in the minds of the judicious, whether the advantages of any given plan, will exceed the expence of carrying it into execution. If we examine the common fields, which are the fubject of this enquiry, we fhall find, that for the moft confiderable part, proprietors who have a property in many hundreds of acres in any parifh, have not more than two or three acres at moft connected together; the refidue lies in acres and half acres, quite disjointed, and tenants under the fame land-owner, crofs each other continually in performing their neceffary daily labour. A general exchange of lands in the refpective parifhes would be a very defirable object, in cafes (if they can poffibly exift) where a general inclofure and divifion could not take place, fo that each man's property would be allotted together in large parcels; by this procedure, at leaft a moiety of the occupier's expences in cultivating the foil might be faved.

General divifions and inclofures of the common fields, are the only means of promoting the good of the country to the utmoft, utmost, by means of which each proprietor will have his property in a contiguous situation; he will be enabled to apply the soil to its right use, (that is to say, the arable land to pasture, and the pasture to arable, as can be best turned to his advantage), to introduce the best systems of agriculture, which are particularly adapted to different soils, to effect a competent drainage, to promote the growth of timber, to bring about an arrangement of tythes so highly desirable for all parties interested in the soil and its productions. And it may be here observed, that the Bishop of LINCOLN has, with very great prudence and judgement, suggested a regulation for a commutation of tythes in his diocese (of which this county is a part) when common fields are inclosed, which is found to answer so well, that it is to be hoped it will be every where adopted. By this plan, the money payments for tithes, vary according to the price of corn from time to time, a procedure equitable towards the land-owners and occupiers, and highly secure for the clergy, because it prevents the abuses which too frequently have befallen the interest of the clergy, in consequence of the mismanagement of the allotments which have been made to them of land, given in lieu of tithes: for it cannot be supposed, that gentlemen, bred up merely in scholastic pursuits, are always competent to let the land they receive, so as to preserve the permanency of its yearly value. It is with pleasure I add, wherever this plan has been carried into effect, it has been attended with the desired success. Those who may be desirous of obtaining further information upon this subject, may consult the regulations in the Act of Parliament lately passed, respecting the inclosing of Milton Bryant, in Bedfordshire, and Tealby, in Lincolnshire.

Inclosed land, managed to the greatest advantage, stands not in need of being folded with sheep when in a state of fallow, by which procedure the produce of the pasture land is laid upon the arable, to which, according to the old system, no return of manure can be made; for under an improved system of hus-

I 2

bandry

bandry, every part of the farm fhould be under fome fpecies of crop, and fallow totally abolifhed, except in thefe inftances; where there any pyrites, metallic, or fulphurous qualities in the foil, in which cafes, being pulverized and turned up to the air, with a proper dreffing of lime, are the only remedies ; but where the drilling and horfe-hoeing hufbandry are purfued, the latter operation fufficiently loofens the foil, and opens the way for the fibres of plants to obtain proper and neceffary nourifhment.

To introduce every argument which might be urged to prove the falutary effects of inclofing commons, common fields and wafte lands, would far exceed the limits of my prefent plan, or the neceffities of the cafe.

It has been obferved, by thofe who are prejudiced in favour of ancient cuftoms and methods, that fome inclofures have not anfwered the expences attending them; but when we confider the plain truth of the matter, it will be found, that mifmanagement and abufe in the mode of bringing about the meafure, as well as the carrying it into effect, has been the true caufe of the ill fuccefs which may have fometimes attended it.

Whoever apprehends, that the occupiers of common fields, are neceffarily tied down to any precife mode management, by the cuftom of any parifh, are grofsly miftaken; for each occupier is only under an obligation to the others, not to break up any of the commonable land, to fet apart the regular field or apportionment of fallow, to open his ditches and water courfes ; not to fuffer the thiftles and weeds to be feeded upon his neighbour; and to ftock the field according to the practice of the parifh. In all other matters he may drive the land, force it totally out of heart; firft, by negligence in fallowing, and next, by fowing wheat upon all his fallowed land, which fhould be divided between barley and wheat, and in fowing oats in fucceffion to wheat and barley, inftead of beans or peafe; and in all this mifmanagement, he does not infringe

upon

upon his brother farmers. But it has frequently occurred to me in practice, that some of the occupiers of a common field, are pursuing the best possible mode of management the situations are capable of, whilst others are reducing land, intermixed therewith, to the lowest state of poverty, beggary, and rubbish, making the respective value of the inheritance to vary three, four, or more years purchase; and upon the inclosure of common fields it frequently occurs, that commissioners are obliged to consider such worn-out land of considerably less value than such parts as have been well farmed; of course, the proprietors, whose misfortune it has been to have their land badly occupied, have had a smaller share, upon the general division of the property, than they otherwise would have had, in case their land had been better farmed.

No drilling, hoeing, or dibbling is pursued in common fields; but in some instances, the sheep are turned into the beans, to eat out a part of the weeds. But this is a miserable substitute for properly hoeing, breaking the fibres of the plants, and occasioning their throwing out fresh ones, thereby destroying weeds, moulding up the plants, and profitably employing and bringing up the infant poor in agricultural pursuits, of which the country stands much in need.

A well digested general bill, for the inclosures of commons, common fields, and waste lands, would wonderfully operate towards the success of inclosures, as it would be a means of saving a very considerable expence in the outset of the business.

It should form a material part of the duty of persons employed as agents for proprietors, whose estates are inclosed, to prevent very expensive buildings from being erected. A profusion of money has been lavished upon useless buildings not requisite for a due occupation of the land, and which is a heavy burden upon the proprietors and occupiers, without answering any good purpose.

It

It has been erroneouffly infifted upon by fome perfons, that certain foils are not adapted for that improved fyftem of hufbandry, which ought to take place upon an inclofure, in order to pay the expences attending it. Strong clayey land with a fhallow ftaple, it is granted will not admit of fo much improvement as other foils, upon which green winter food may be produced in perfection, as turnips, cole, or rape feed, or cabbages; and where the drill hufbandry, under a proper courfe of ameliorating crops, (as peafe, beans, and other pulfe, interwoven with a rotation of white grain crops, and artificial graffes in fucceffion) are judicioufly purfued, It is alfo certain, that mixed foil, light loamy, fandy, and gravelly foils, if they are in a ftate of common field, anfwer beft to the proprietors upon an inclofure; fuch foils having been farmed according to the ancient common-field hufbandry, are very weak, poor, foul, and unproductive. The quick repetitions of the fame forts of grain, and the too frequently breaking and turning over the foil, already too light, tends to let the mucilage be wafhed away, and to efcape the reach of the roots of the grain; which difadvantages are to be remedied, in a great degree, upon an introduction of an improved fyftem of hufbandry. Strong clayey land, with a fhallow ftaple, may be very much improved by means of an inclofure, upon which a complete drainage may be effected, wheat, beans, artificial graffes, &c. cultivated to perfection; thus promoting more abundantly the means of improving and fupporting cattle and fheep, and very much meliorating their water layer; and in many inftances, on fuch land green winter food may be produced, as cole, rape, or cabbages, where manure in pretty ftrong dreffings can be afforded for that purpofe.

THE

THE BREED OF NEAT CATTLE,

———

By means of a general inclosure, may be improved at least 40 per cent. and supported upon the same weight of aliment as they are now.

The SHEEP may be improved in their carcases at least 10s. each, and in their fleeces three shillings per fleece, in like manner, and under the like circumstances.

———

TIMBER AND UNDERWOOD,

———

Which derives its support from below the superstratum of soil, and not dependent upon it, may, in many instances, be planted with great success upon land which is of very low quality, for any of the purposes of cultivation.

Whenever underwood is cut, the sorts ought to be particularly examined, and such as are unproductive or unprofitable, grubbed up, and other sorts planted in their stead ; the same care should be used in selecting, planting, preserving, and cultivating timber best adapted to their respective soils.

IMPROVEMENT

OF

INCLOSED ARABLE AND PASTURE LAND.

THE application of foil to its right ufe, is a matter of the utmoft importance to the kingdom in general, but more particularly to the landed intereft. It will be found, upon due enquiry, that a very confiderable quantity of land, which is now pafture, cannot be improved without its being firft brought into an arable ftate; and it will be alfo found, (though in inftances more rare) that certain parts now arable, might be better applied to the purpofes of pafture.

It certainly requires fome judgment, to make the neceffary difcrimination, and to draw covenants between landlord and tenant, for the regulation of the fyftem, and due care muft be taken to fee them enforced. For want of competent judgment in perfons employed in fuch concerns, or from neglect, abufes have frequently happened, and felf-interefted tenants have plowed up pafture land, without attending to any improvement; but on the contrary, have continued to crop the land with grain whilft it would produce any, and afterwards it has fallen into the landlord's hands in a reduced ftate; from fuch circumftances the proprietors became alarmed, and have rather preferred that their land fhould continue in a ftate of perpetual pafture, than that it fhould be converted to arable,

under

under a rifque of its being exhaufted; and prejudice againſt the plough is fo very ſtrong, that it is not unuſual to meet with perſons in the habit of acting as furveyors, who eſtimate the value of land, merely in proportion as it may be confidered adapted for being laid down in paſture. I am confident that due proportions of paſture and arable land, beſt anſwer the purpoſes of an occupier; and according to the ſize of a farm, fo ought theſe proportions to be laid out, by which means green winter food for feeding cattle and ſheep, and ſtraw for litter is provided; and manure ariſing therefrom may be afforded to be laid upon the paſtures, whilſt, by a judicious ſyſtem of agriculture, the arable land will, in a very great degree, ſupport itſelf in high condition.

It is no advantage for an occupier to be permitted to uſe the plough, unleſs he can have a ſufficient quantity of arable land, to carry him on ſyſtematically for green winter food, &c·

It is a common practice where plowing is permitted, to ſuffer tenants to break up certain portions of paſture land under agreements, to lay ſuch land down again for paſture at ſtipulated times, and then to break up other parts, ſuch land is generally impoveriſhed when it is laid down, and ever afterwards it continues unproductive in that ſtate.

Farms confiſting wholly of paſture and meadow land, muſt neceſſarily be impoveriſhed, becauſe a certain quantity muſt be every year mown, and an adequate return of manure cannot be made for the injury done by the ſcythe.

Meadow land upon the banks of rivers, which may be occaſionally watered, and very rich paſture land in low ſituations, cannot be more profitably applied; but paſture land of inferior quality, and more eſpecially ſuch as has been injudiciouſly plowed, and improperly laid down, may be converted to more profitable purpoſes, by plowing, and introducing the improved ſyſtem of huſbandry; at leaſt a third of the produce of every acre of paſture land, as often as it is renewed, is waſted by the ſoil of the animals which depaſture on it. When gentle-

K   men

men of landed property shall attend more to agriculture, and grasses shall be better understood, and the most valuable sort selected, we shall have very little land permanently under pasture, such grasses will be cultivated in like manner to lucern, and cattle and sheep will probably be most profitably stall fed; a practice intitled to consideration and experiment. But whilst any land is used as pasture or meadow, it ought to be improved to the utmost it is capable of, by levelling the ant-hills, draining, manuring, rolling, &c.

The best mode of levelling the ant-hills is, by cutting every third hill annually, and spreading its contents, and laying down the sod upon its base, (provided it is of a good sort of grass, if not, to sow grass seeds theron), by which means the whole business will be performed in three years, and the land will not be overburthened at any time with too much dead soil. In other cases it may be adviseable, upon poor clayey land, to cut up the ant-hills and carry them off; or, in desperate cases, to plow the whole. Much depends upon the particular cases, and a man of judgement will act accordingly.

Whether a farm consists of land which has been long in tillage, or land converted from pasture to arable, the most approved system of agriculture, best adapted to the soil, ought to be applied: which, considered in a general way, is, by keeping off successions of white grain, (viz. wheat, barley, rye, and oats), to interweave meliorating crops alternately between crops of white grain; to drain, drill, hoe, weed, and preserve each sort; to lay down for a certain time with grass seeds, such parts as shall in any previous year have produced turnips, cole seed, or cabbages, with the next crop of grain, for one or more years. Thus stock of every description may be improved to the utmost the soil is capable of maintaining, which will be best carried into effect, by an equal regard in selecting the best sorts, and in the care which is taken in cultivating the means for its support.

A ju-

A judicious agent can easily draw covenants adapted to every improvement the soil is capable of, giving the occupier full scope for doing well, and preventing him from injuring the property he occupies; and thus, the great objection of granting leases, without which no general improvement can be expected, is effectually removed.

IMPROVEMENT

IN

MEADOW LAND.

It has been already remarked, that the Ouze is the principal river which runs though this county; along its banks is a considerable quantity of rich meadow land, which is subject to be overflowed at all seasons of the year. When the water comes down from Buckinghamshire with any considerable rapidity, it frequently happens, that the crops of hay are either considerably damaged, or totally carried away. The water, which might be made a source of great advantage, is, in the present state of things, an evil of no small magnitude. A considerable number of water-mills are placed upon this

stream

ftream, which ferve to increafe the rifque or damage, and more efpecially as the conftruction of their wheels are not generally on the improved plan; and as there is no certain gauge or level generally obferved, to which the water fhall be held up, nor any pofitive laws enforced for throwing open flood gates upon the approach of an increafed quantity of water— I propofe, that either the water mills fhould be taken away, or under a general or particular Act of Parliament, the river fhould where neceffary be widened, and embanked in a competent manner; that the land-owners fhould have a power of taking water out of the river, at certain times and feafons, to water the meadows, when it may be done with the leaft injury to the mills; that all flood gates and wafte water fhould be regulated in an efficient manner, fo that in times of flood, or when the banks of the river are overflowed, the water may fpeedily make its exit, without being in any degree dependant on the mills.

The expence of carrying this plan into execution would be inconfiderable, when compared with the advantages attending it. The foil which will neceffarily be taken from the nooks and corners of the land, or from the fides of the river, to widen it, in order more effectually to carry off the floods, will ferve to embank it: and when this bufinefs is performed, the meadows may be drained where neceffary; the crops of hay and eddifh may at all times be preferved; and the water, which is now the dread of the occupiers, may be made the fource of a moft invaluable improvement, by judicioufly watering the land.

A tax may be laid upon the land thus to be improved, in proportion to the yearly value of the improvement, or of the mills to be taken away, or any other expences attending the plan, which will be but a fmall drawback upon the advantages to be derived from an immediate improvement of the meadows, of perhaps twenty fhillings per acre.

ON

or

IMPROVING THE SITUATION OF THE LABOURER.

━━━━━

COMFORTABLE habitations fhould be provided upon every eftate, for the induftrious labourers who are emp'oyed upon it; and where it is neceffary that any new erections fhall take place, I would recommend, that they fhould be placed contiguous to each other, from which circumftance the conduct of each individual would be known to his neighbours; and giving each labourer a portion of land to fupply him with efculen roots, and (where neceffary) with the means of maintaining a hardy cow, of the Scotch or Welch breeds; provifions, thus made for the neceffary labourers upon each eftate, there would be no doubt of an increafe of inhabitants, whofe duty as well as intereft it would be, to exert themfelves to the utmoft of their power for the farmers at all feafons of the year, whilft the influence of the neighbouring magiftracy would be a barrier againft their being oppreffed.

If thefe meafures were to be purfued, and the farmers were provident (as is the cafe in Norfolk and Suffolk) to engage a competent number of labourers, mechanics, artificers, tradefmen, and others, (fome confiderable time before harveft) to affift in the neceffary bufinefs of it, difficulties, loffes, and extraordinary expences, would be in almoft every cafe prevented.

CON-

CONCLUSION.

On the whole, if under the patronage of so valuable an inftitution as the Board of Agriculture, proper meafures were fpeedily taken for the improvement of the county of Bedford, there can be no doubt, that in the fpace of a very few years the population of the county would be confiderably increafed, the fituation of every individual in it would be materially bettered, and the kingdom at large would receive a very important acceffion to its opulence and ftrength.

THE END.

CPSIA information can be obtained at www.ICGtesting.com
Printed in the USA
LVOW02s0105160913

352568LV00005B/169/P